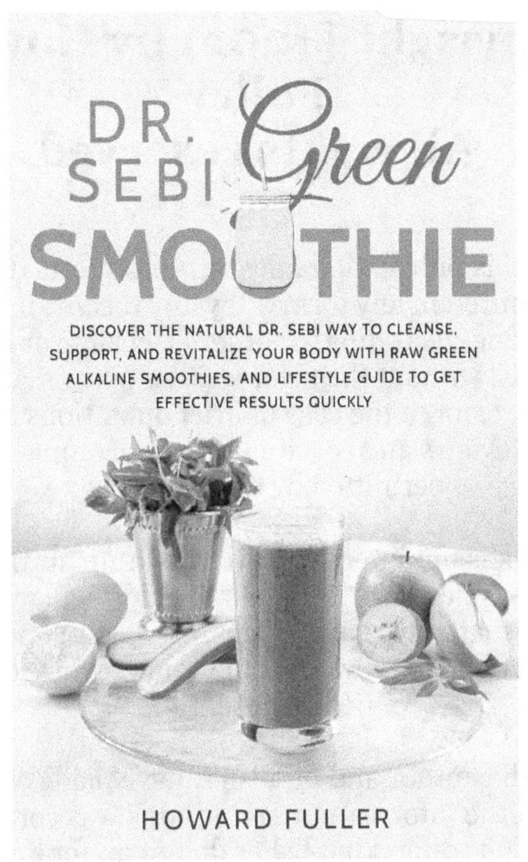


# Dr. Sebi Green Smoothie:
## Discover the Natural Dr. Sebi Way to Cleanse, Support, and Revitalize Your Body with Raw Green Alkaline Smoothies, and Lifestyle Guide to Get Effective Results Quickly

# Table of Content


Table of Content

Introduction

Chapter 1: Get to Know the Benefits
      Who is Dr.Sebi?
      The Plant-Based Healing Process
      Interesting Facts
      What is Dr. Sebi Smoothie Diet?
      Embark Your Weight Loss Journey
      Alter the Microbiome
      Reduce Risk of Diseases
      Rejuvenate Your Body

Chapter 2: Learn More About Green Alkaline Smoothies
      Are They Healthy?
      Understand Body PH
      Increasing the Alkalinity
      Why Can Greens Do Wonders?
      Are there any Risks?
      Foods Approved by Dr. Sebi
      Fruits
      Vegetables
      Nuts & Seeds
      Spices
      Herbal Teas
      Oils

Chapter 3: Adapt Habits to Make a Difference

Drink Lots of Water
Say "NO" to Microwave
Don't Use the Word "Cheat"
Have a Game Plan for Outings
Practice Patience
Plan, Plan, Plan
Prepare - A Smoothie Diet Chart
Stock Your Pantry for a Healthy Diet
Experiment with Your Food
Reward Yourself
Track and Monitor Your Progress

Chapter 4: Foods to Avoid
Canned Fruits or Vegetables
Non-Vegetarian Foods
Fortified & Processed Foods
Dairy
Alcohol
Fried Foods
Fish
Soy Products

Chapter 5: Keep Keep Going After the Smoothie Cleanse
Gradually Add More Foods
Stick to Healthy Foods
Chew Slowly
Avoid Overeating
Hydration is the key
Remember Your End Goals

Chapter 6: Dr. Sebi 17 Approved Alkaline Green Smoothies
Sea Moss Apple Smoothie
Avocado Green Smoothie
Moringa Apple Smoothie
Cucumber Apple Smoothie

Wild Kale Apple Smoothie
Carrot Apple Smoothie with Ginger, Turmeric and Cardamom
Cucumber Lime Smoothie
Tomato Ginger Apple Smoothie
Avocado Strawberry Green Smoothie
Papaya Green Smoothie
Orange Green Smoothie With Ginger
Passion Fruit Green Smoothie
Spinach Apple Green Smoothie
Raspberry Green Smoothie
Celery Green Smoothie
Banana Celery Green Smoothie
Grapefruit Green Smoothie

Conclusion

Thank You

Other Books By Author

About Author

# Introduction

If you are reading this, you must have a sincere desire to be healthy. There are many health books out there, but how many of them can help you achieve this desire?

This book is different from the rest! It is a compilation of over 40 years of knowledge and experience from Dr. Sebi. The reader will learn about how to achieve true health and healing with green smoothies.

Dr. Sebi was a world-renowned scientist, herbalist, and healer. He had a degree in Medicine from Central America University located in Los Angeles, California. Dr. Sebi has been featured on many national television programs all over the world and has appeared on the front page of The New York Times. Dr. Sebi's knowledge can help the world to heal and this book is one of the best ways to show you how he did it!

This book is broken down into 6 simple chapters, each focusing on a different aspect of Dr. Sebi's green smoothie program. The reader will learn about the importance of eating your greens, how to prepare your greens for maximum absorption, how to choose the right greens for your body, how to combine your green smoothies for maximum effect, how to make sure your body is absorbing the nutrients you put in it, and much more!

Dr. Sebi's green smoothie program is not just about making a green smoothie every morning. Dr. Sebi was an intelligent man and he knew that there was a lot more to his green smoothie recipe than just throwing some greens into a blender with water and drinking it down. He knew that he had to prepare his greens in the right way so that his body would be able to absorb all of their nutrients. Dr. Sebi's green smoothie program is the culmination of over 40 years of knowledge and experience into one simple book!

 This book will help you achieve true health and healing with Dr. Sebi's Green Smoothie Program!

# Chapter 1

# Get to Know the Benefits

Have you heard of the green smoothies? If you haven't, then you are in for a great treat. Green smoothies are great drinks that have numerous health benefits. This is what makes them unique from other drinks. The great thing about these smoothies is that they can be used to treat various medical conditions. For this reason, many people have been using them to treat diseases such as diabetes and cancer. In this chapter, we will look at the various benefits that come with green smoothies.

Dr. Sebi has been in the health industry for a long time. In fact, he has come up with some of the best ways to treat different ailments. One of his most famous ways is through green smoothies. These smoothies are made up of plant-based ingredients and are meant to help people treat various diseases and ailments.

Let's take a look at the various benefits of green smoothies.

## Who is Dr.Sebi?

Dr. Sebi was born in Honduras, and he went to the United States to study medicine. He is a great doctor who has helped numerous people with their health problems. This is why he is known as the herbalist doctor. He has also been recognized by different people for his great work.

The reason why Dr. Sebi became famous was due to his herbal medicine that had helped many people. In fact, he has been able to help those people who had terminal illnesses such as cancer. This is because he didn't use any pharmaceuticals. Instead, he used natural herbs that could help people treat their health problems.

This is why Dr. Sebi has become famous in the health industry. He has helped a lot of people to be healthy again. The great thing about his herbal medicine is that it treats various diseases and ailments without causing any side effects. This is why his methods are considered to be effective and safe by many people.

The green smoothies that Dr. Sebi created are natural drinks that you can use to treat different medical conditions. If you want to learn more about these green smoothies, then keep reading this chapter because we will look at the benefits of these smoothies in detail here.

## The Plant-Based Healing Process

Dr. Sebi has come up with some of the best ways to treat various ailments in the world. The great thing about his methods is that they are natural and safe. In fact, you will not get any side effects when you decide to use his herbal medicine. The reason why he uses herbal medicine is that he wants to help people who are suffering from chronic diseases such as diabetes and cancer.

He does this by looking at the root cause of the disease or ailment. When it comes to treating problems such as cancer, Dr. Sebi relies on plants that have medicinal properties. These plants have been used for centuries to treat various ailments in Africa and other parts of the world. Some of these plants include aloe vera, goji berry, and coconut oil among others.

Dr. Sebi has looked into these plants in great detail so that he can find out how they can be used to treat different health conditions. He was able to come up with some great methods that you can use at home as well as through a clinical treatment program that he offers for those who need it more urgently than others. We will look at how these smoothies work shortly. However, before we do so, let's take a look at some of the benefits that come with them.

## Interesting Facts

The great thing about green smoothies is that they have numerous benefits. These benefits have been proven by numerous studies that have been conducted on them. Here are some of the benefits that come with the green smoothies.

**1.They can help people lose weight**

If you want to lose weight, then you should consider using Dr Sebi's green smoothies. This is because they are made up of fruits and vegetables which are low in calories and fat content. This means that you will get enough nutrients from these drinks but they will not make you gain weight. The great thing about these drinks is that they contain more antioxidants than other drinks such as coffee or tea, meaning that they can be used to remove harmful toxins from your body and even improve your body's immune system function.

**2.They can decrease the risk of diabetes**

Green smoothies are low in sugar content which makes them a good choice for those who suffer from diabetes or those who have a family history of diabetes. In case your family suffers from diabetes, then you should consider using Dr Sebi's green smoothies to help prevent yourself from suffering from this condition as well. If used regularly, his smoothies can help in maintaining the blood sugar levels in your body.

### 3. They can improve your vision

In case you are suffering from glaucoma or cataracts, then you can use Dr Sebi's green smoothies to improve your vision. This is because they contain rich amounts of beta-carotene which is an important nutrient for the eyes. Other ingredients such as spinach and avocado are also good for improving the eye health of people using them.

### 4. They can improve your digestive system

If you have problems with your digestion system, then you should consider using Dr Sebi's green smoothies. This is because they contain high amounts of fiber which can help in opening up your bowels and removing toxins from your body. In fact, the fiber content in these drinks will help eliminate constipation and other bowel problems.

### 5. They can improve the immune system

Dr Sebi uses a lot of natural ingredients that can boost the immune system in your body. These ingredients are also great for improving the blood circulation in your body which helps to remove any toxins from it. By using his smoothies, you will be able to get rid of harmful toxins that may have accumulated in your body over time. This is because they contain a lot of antioxidants that will help to protect your body from diseases and infections.

### 6. They can treat cancer

Dr Sebi's green smoothies are known for their anti-cancer properties. In fact, they are considered to be one of the best ways to prevent cancer in those who use them regularly. Some of these ingredients include cinnamon, astragalus root, flax seed oil among others which are known for their anti-cancer properties. If you want to protect yourself from cancer, then you should consider using Dr Sebi's green smoothies.

### 7. They can boost brain function

Dr Sebi's green smoothies can also be used to improve the overall function of your brain. This is because they contain a lot of nutrients that will help boost your memory and enhance the functioning of your brain cells in general. By using these drinks regularly, you will be able to get rid of any memory problems that you have been having over time. You will also be able to improve your mental clarity as well as focus when it comes to using these drinks regularly.

## What is Dr. Sebi Smoothie Diet?

The green smoothies are plant-based drinks that you can make at home. The great thing about them is that they are easy to prepare. In fact, you will not need to use any special tools or appliances to do so. You only have to follow the recipe carefully and you will be able to make great drinks in no time at all.

As we have mentioned above, these smoothies are made from natural ingredients and they will help relieve your symptoms without causing any side effects. The great thing about them is that they can be used for different medical conditions such as diabetes, cancer, and obesity among others. This is why Dr Sebi has come up with these great recipes for you.

**The Secret Behind These Smoothies:**

When it comes to the secret behind these drinks, Dr Sebi combines a combination of various foods and ingredients together in order to make the best smoothie for you. For instance, if you want a drink that can help treat cancer, then he will look into what kind of ingredients will fight cancer effectively. He then combines them together in a specific way so that they can be used for treating this ailment properly. The good thing about his methods is that they work effectively and naturally without causing any side effects.

**The Great Taste:**

Most people think that these green smoothies are meant to help them lose weight and fight diseases. However, this isn't the case at all. In fact, you will find these drinks to taste great. This is because Dr Sebi has made sure that the ingredients taste great when used in a specific combination. He has come up with some of the best recipes for you so that you can make your own smoothie easily without worrying about anything else.

## Embark Your Weight Loss Journey

Greens are great ingredients that you can use to lose weight. This is because they are very healthy for the body. In fact, they contain various nutrients that will help you to lose weight. For this reason, it is very important for people to include green as part of their diets.

Green smoothies are great drinks because they are made up of green vegetables and fruits. They are healthy, and they can help you lose a lot of weight in a short time. Not only that but these drinks will also recharge your body with energy. This is why it is important for you to add them in your diet if you want to lose weight easily and effectively.

This is what makes green smoothies useful for people who want to lose weight quickly and safely. They are healthy, and they can be added into your regular diet without causing any problems at all. In fact, these smoothies have been recognized by many people who have used them before, and now they have become fans of the drink as well.

## Alter the Microbiome

The microbiome is known as the collection of bacteria and yeast located in the gut. The great thing about this microbiome is that it helps to improve the health of a person by breaking down food and absorbing vitamins and minerals. It is essential to maintain good health, and this is why you need to ensure that it remains healthy.

This is why green smoothies are great because they can help to restore the microbiome. They do this by providing people with probiotics that they can use to boost their gut health. This is why green smoothies are considered useful for treating diseases such as diarrhea, constipation, inflammatory bowel disease, irritable bowel syndrome and leaky gut syndrome.

This means that green smoothies have numerous benefits because they can be used to treat various diseases. You can use them to treat different medical conditions without having any side effects.

## Reduce Risk of Diseases

Green smoothies are great drinks that you can use to improve the health of your body. They are not just good for treating certain diseases, but they can also help people reduce their risk of getting sick. This is because they are packed with nutrients. The great thing about these nutrients is that they help to improve the general health of a person.

One example is vitamin C which is an antioxidant that helps to prevent heart disease and cancer. Another example is vitamin A which plays an important role in maintaining healthy eyes and skin. In fact, it also helps to protect against cancer and heart diseases. Green smoothies also contain antioxidants such as beta-carotene and lycopene which promote a healthy heart and eyesight.

The best thing about green smoothies is that they can be used to prevent numerous diseases such as heart disease, cancer, diabetes and many more conditions. This makes them great drinks that you can use to treat various medical conditions without using any pharmaceuticals or surgery.

## Rejuvenate Your Body

No matter what your age is, you will benefit from using green smoothies. This is because they can help to improve the health of your body. They are great drinks that can help you to get rid of the feeling of fatigue and help you to feel energized.

They also help to improve the digestion system, leading to better health. They can also help you sleep better at night, which is essential for a healthy life.

The ingredients used in green smoothies are great for the body. This is because they help to improve the general health of a person. The best thing about these ingredients is that they have numerous nutrients that help to keep your body healthy. The great thing about green smoothies is that they can be used to treat several conditions without having any side effects.

# Chapter 2

# Learn More About Green Alkaline Smoothies

Green alkaline smoothies are a great way to alkalize your body. As we know, the body is built with a pH of about 7.365. The body functions best within a pH of 7.365 or slightly above or below that number. Green alkaline smoothies are used to alkalize the body only when it is extremely acidic, which results in illness and many degenerative diseases. These illnesses include cancer, diabetes, heart disease and even osteoporosis. We do not recommend eating green alkaline smoothies on a daily basis because most people do not believe in drinking their vegetables and thus they will be deprived of nutrients that they need from vegetables.

In this chapter, we will discuss some of the health benefits of green alkaline smoothies. Some of these health benefits and some of the risks associated with green alkaline smoothies will be discussed. We will also discuss some of the health benefits that can be achieved by drinking these green alkaline smoothies on a daily basis.

## Are They Healthy?

The main goal of green alkaline smoothies is to alkalize the body. They are able to accomplish this goal because they are filled with vegetables and fruits. These vegetables and fruits are filled with nutrients that have been proven to alkalize the body. The following list is a sample of some of these vegetables and fruits.

Dr. Sebi's Green Alkaline Smoothie is shown to be a great way to alkalize the body. It is also a good way to detoxify the body and get rid of many of those toxic substances.

## Understand Body PH

A body's pH is a measurement of the acidity or alkalinity of the blood. The body functions best within a pH of 7.365 or slightly above or below that number. The body will become ill and degenerative diseases will occur when the pH is too acidic or too alkaline.

The best way to keep the body in balance is by eating a balanced diet. The body can become too acidic or alkaline because of the foods we eat. Some foods are acidic and some are alkaline. Some foods have a pH of about 7.365 and some have a pH of about 4.4, which is extremely alkaline and some have an extremely high acidic pH of about 1, which is extremely acidic.

Drinking green alkaline smoothies on a daily basis helps to alkalize your body and it can help prevent the diseases that occur when the body becomes too acidic or too alkaline. This will also help to minimize the risk of getting sick and help your body to stay in balance.

## Increasing the Alkalinity

When the body becomes too acidic or when it is extremely acidic, it is at risk of getting sick and the body cannot function properly. Green alkaline smoothies help to alkalize your body.

It is important to note that the body will become too acidic as a result of eating too many acidic foods. Eating alkaline foods will help to alkalize the body and minimize the risk of getting sick.

For example, an unhealthy diet can cause the body to become too acidic. If a person eats too many carbohydrates, it will make them sick and they will develop metabolic syndrome. This is a condition that causes the body to become too acidic.

Other foods that will make the body acidic are dairy products, fried foods and sugar. These foods will increase the risk of getting sick because they are extremely acidic and they cannot be digested properly.

Green alkaline smoothies can alkalize your body by eating alkaline foods that are good for health. These green alkaline smoothies help to increase the pH of your blood and this helps to balance your body out. Green alkaline smoothies will help to minimize the risk of getting sick by improving your health. They can also prevent degenerative diseases that occur when a person has too many toxins in their body.

## Why Can Greens Do Wonders?

According to the studies that have been done by Dr. Sebi and many other doctors, vegetables have a special property that makes them alkaline. These properties are called anti-oxidants and when consumed on a daily basis they can have a good effect on the body as they can alkalize the body. Green smoothies are made from vegetables with these antioxidants. When you consume these green smoothies, they will be absorbed by your body as nutrients. As we know, the vegetables that we consume are macro-nutrients in nature because they are very large and thus too much of them is not good for the body. When the body receives too much of these macronutrients, it tends to store some of them as fat. This is why you should consume green smoothies in moderation because if you drink them in excess, you can gain unwanted weight.

These greens help to alkalize your body because they contain a large amount of chlorophyll which is an antioxidant. When a person consumes too much sugar or fat, then their bodies become acidic because sugar and fat are acid forming in nature; this results in illnesses such as diabetes and cancer.

Some studies show that green smoothies have helped people with diabetes to reduce their blood sugar levels. It is recommended that people with diabetes should consume about 5 cups of greens per day. This will help them to alkalize their bodies and reduce the amount of sugar in their bloodstreams.

Other studies show that green smoothies have helped people who have cancer to alkalize their bodies. These green smoothies help to oxygenate the body and thus there is high metabolism, and this results in the destruction of cancer cells.

For example, one of these studies was done by Dr. Sebi who has helped many cancer patients to alkalize their bodies. He has also helped many people to get rid of diabetes and other degenerative diseases. He had a patient who had cancer, but after he started consuming green smoothies he noticed that his cancer disappeared within a few months.

## Are there any Risks?

Yes, there are some risks associated with green smoothies. One of the main risks is that if people consume too much green smoothies, it can be bad for their health. People should not overuse these vegetables simply because they may contain harmful substances such as pesticides. This is why Dr. Sebi has recommended that people should grow their own vegetables at home or go to their local farmers and buy locally grown vegetables without using any pesticides. You can also buy organic vegetables from your local stores, but you need to read the labels very carefully before you buy them because some of these organic vegetables may have been imported from other countries and they may contain some pesticides in them.

Another risk associated with green smoothies are the microorganisms in the vegetables. You need to wash your vegetables well before you consume them and if you use a blender, make sure that you clean it well before using it again. Some people use a blender then wash it without cleaning it very well; this results in cross-contamination and this is a major problem when you consume these green smoothies every day.

Some people who do not like eating greens may dislike drinking green alkaline smoothies because they have never tasted them before. They may think that they will taste very bitter, but they do not. You can sweeten them up with some fruits and some other sweeteners if you need to.

## Foods Approved by Dr. Sebi

Dr. Sebi has approved very specific foods that are to be used for his green alkaline smoothies. He does not recommend that you use any other than these foods. The following is a list of the foods that are approved by Dr. Sebi.

## Fruits

### 1.Limes

Limes are a great green alkaline smoothie fruit to use. They are very acidic, being at a pH of 2 or 3, but when mixed with other vegetables and a little lemon juice, they will turn alkaline. They are also quite sour which helps to ensure that the body is properly hydrated by balancing the pH of the body.

### 2.Apples

Apple juice is a great green alkaline smoothie fruit to use. It is acidic in nature, but it is also very sweet which helps to balance out the pH of the smoothie if it is not sour enough. Apples are also great for alkalizing the body as well as for healing many diseases such as arthritis, diabetes and obesity. Apples are also great for reducing acidity in the body and making it more alkaline.

### 3.Pears

Pears are another green alkaline smoothie fruit that should be used when making these smoothies, but they should be used sparingly because of their high sugar content which can cause a person to gain weight if they drink too much of them or too frequently. They are best used when mixed with other vegetables or fruits that are more sour and acidic in nature.

## 4.Mangos

Mangoes are a great green alkaline smoothie fruit to use. They are acidic in nature, but they are also very sweet which helps to balance the pH of the smoothie. They are also great for reducing acidity in the body and making it more alkaline. The high sugar content of mangos can cause weight gain if you drink them too much or too frequently, so they should be used sparingly when making green alkaline smoothies.

## 5.Papayas

Papayas are a great green alkaline smoothie fruit to use because they are both sour and sweet which means that they balance the pH of the body when consumed with other fruits that have enough acidity to balance it out. It is one of the best fruits that can be used for making green alkaline smoothies because it is very high in water, fiber, nutrients and enzymes which help to keep your body hydrated, cleansed and healthy. It is also great for reducing acidity in the body and making it more alkaline. Papayas also contain many different kinds of antioxidants that help your body stay healthy while fighting off many diseases.

## 6.Grapefruits

Grapefruits are a tangy fruit that has a very strong scent. They can be eaten in its entirety, including its skin. The grapefruit is one of the most powerful fruits in the world and has been used in many products that are sold in health food stores. Grapefruits are a great source of vitamin C, and they also have a high concentration of beta carotene. This fruit can protect your cells from free radicals that can cause cancer, and it can lower your risk of heart disease.

## 7.Bananas

Bananas are a good source of vitamins and minerals, making it a perfect fruit for your smoothie. It also has natural sugars that are good to make your smoothie a little sweeter. Bananas also give you a healthy dose of energy to keep you going throughout the day.

## 8.Blueberries

Blueberries are another perfect fruit for your smoothie because of their high antioxidant content and low sugar content. They are also rich in fiber and have been shown to help with cardiovascular health by reducing the risk of strokes and heart attacks. You can use blueberries in any type of smoothie but if you plan on using it with vegetables or greens to make a green smoothie, then it would be best if you use organic blueberries to prevent pesticides from getting into your system.

## 9.Cherries

Cherries are considered a superfood because of its antioxidant content. It also helps to lower the risk of cardiovascular disease and it is also good for your skin. Cherries have a high amount of vitamin C, Potassium, Iron and Calcium. It also has a high amount of fiber so it can help you feel full longer.

## 10.Oranges

Oranges are a sweet and tangy fruit. They are rich in antioxidants and vitamin C. Oranges also have a high amount of fiber so it helps you feel full for a longer period of time. It also has vitamin A, B6 and Folate to help your body stay healthy and it is also good for your skin. Oranges can be added to any smoothie but it goes especially well with green smoothies because of its tanginess and sweetness.

## 11. Coconuts

Coconuts are a versatile fruit. It can be eaten as a snack, added to any smoothie or used as an ingredient in baking or cooking. It also has a lot of health benefits which makes it popular and easy to find in grocery stores. Coconut has a high amount of potassium and fiber, so it can help you feel full for longer periods of time. It also contains vitamin C which is essential for your immune system and keeping you healthy. Coconut also contains a good source of protein which can help you feel more full.

## 12. Prunes

Prunes are a dried plum that can help you lose weight. They are also known to help with constipation and bad breath. Prunes are also very high in fiber which helps you feel full for longer periods of time. Prunes are also rich in antioxidants to help you fight off diseases and they can help lower cholesterol levels.

## 13. Grapes

Grapes contain a high amount of antioxidants, potassium, vitamin C and fiber. It also has a low sugar content and its sweetness is considered a natural sugar that is good for your body. Grapes are another fruit that goes well with any smoothie or juice you want to drink because it has a sweet taste and it gives your smoothie some texture as well as flavor. Grapes can be easily found in most grocery stores but when selecting grapes make sure to get organic as they have the highest antioxidant content when they are organic, compared to conventional grapes.

### 14.Peaches

Peaches are another sweet fruit that is perfect for your smoothie. Peaches have a high amount of antioxidant content and a good source of potassium. It is also a good source of calcium, vitamin C, and fiber.

### 15.Melons

Melons are mostly made up of water, making them a good fruit for your smoothie. They can help you stay hydrated and they are also good for your skin. Melons also have a high amount of potassium and fiber. They are also sweet so they can help sweeten your smoothie.

### 16.Soursops

Soursops are a very good source of vitamins and minerals, making it a great fruit for weight loss. They also have powerful antioxidants that can help you keep your immune system strong. They are great for those who have high cholesterol levels.

### 17.Dates

Dates are a very good source of minerals and vitamins that are good for you. They have a lot of nutritional benefits that help you lose weight and keep your immune system strong. They also have natural sugars that can make your smoothie sweeter without adding any extra sugar. They are also great for people who are trying to stop smoking because they help curb the cravings. Dates also help keep your skin looking beautiful and reduce the appearance of wrinkles.

## 18.Raisins

Raisins are a fruit made of dehydrated grapes. They are high in sugar, but that's what makes it so great. It can be used to sweeten your smoothie without adding any extra sugar. It is also a good source of fiber, iron and zinc.

## 19.Raspberries

Raspberries are great for your skin as they contain anti-aging properties that will make you look young and beautiful. It is also a good source of antioxidants that can help you maintain your immune system and keep you from getting sick. They are also great for your cardiovascular health as they contain omega-3 fatty acids.

## 20.Figs

Figs are fruits that are great for weight loss. They contain a good amount of fiber and water, making them great for weight loss. They also have a lot of vitamins and minerals that are good for your health.

## 21.Prunes

Prunes are fruits that are good for weight loss. They have a lot of fiber, making them a great choice for weight loss. They also have a lot of potassium that can help lower your blood pressure as well as sugars and vitamins and minerals to keep you healthy.

## 22.Tamarinds

Tamarinds are a good source of vitamins and minerals, making it a great fruit for weight loss. It is great for slowing down the absorption of sugars into your bloodstream. They also contain a lot of fiber that can help you lose weight.

### 23.Pomegranate

Pomegranates are great for weight loss as they have a lot of fiber. They also have a good amount of nitrates that are good for your cardiovascular health as well as anti-inflammatory properties that can help you lose weight. They are also great for hair growth and skin health.

## Vegetables

### 1.Spinach

Spinach is a very powerful green that is rich in chlorophyll. It is the richest natural source of iron and also contains over 45 different nutrients. It is high in antioxidants, including quercetin, beta carotene and zeaxanthin which are great for our eyesight.

### 2.Kale

Kale is another very popular green that has been around for centuries and has many health benefits. This green contains vitamins A, C, E and K as well as minerals such as calcium, copper, iron, magnesium and manganese. This vegetable has been known to improve our eyesight and can even lower blood pressure.

### 3.Dandelion Greens

Dandelion greens are loaded with calcium, potassium and vitamin A which helps to improve your eyesight too! This green also has anti-inflammatory properties which can help ease certain aches you may be experiencing from time to time.

## 4.Red/Purple Romaine Lettuce

Romaine lettuce is a dark leafy green that is full of vitamin A as well as B vitamins such as folate, riboflavin and thiamin which help to regulate your nervous system function! This green also contains potassium and can help to lower blood pressure.

## 5.Mustard Greens

This green has been used in traditional Chinese medicine for many years and is full of vitamins A and C as well as calcium, iron and magnesium! These nutrients not only help fight inflammation, but they also improve blood circulation.

## 6.Watercress

Watercress is a spicy green that is loaded with vitamin A as well as minerals including calcium, potassium and magnesium! This green has also been shown to lower levels of cholesterol in our bodies which can decrease the risk of heart disease.

## 7.Collard Greens (Black)

Collard greens are a very popular variety of green that can be found in many different recipes from around the world. This green is a great source of calcium as well as vitamins A and C, which are essential for your eyesight. Collard greens also contain anti-inflammatory properties.

## 8.Basil

This green is something that I love to grow in my garden and I add it to many of my recipes! Basil is a common herb used in Italian cuisine but it also has many health benefits! It contains vitamins A, C and K along with many minerals that will help to improve your vision. This green is also anti-inflammatory and can help ease any aches you may feel from time to time! If you don't grow basil at home, you can find this green at many local farmers markets or grocery stores!

## 9.Celery

Celery is a very popular green that is extremely versatile. It can be added to many recipes and even enjoyed on its own! Celery is full of vitamins A, C, K and B-complex vitamins as well as many minerals. This green has been shown to lower blood pressure as well!

## 10.Chard

This green is best when prepared by sautéing or steaming it but it can be eaten raw too! Chard is loaded with vitamin A, along with many minerals such as calcium and magnesium which are essential for our eyesight! This green has also been shown to lower cholesterol levels which decreases the risk of heart disease.

## 11.Avocado

Avocados are very high in fat, but that's what makes it so great. They are also a good source of fiber, vitamins and minerals such as vitamin B6, Potassium, Magnesium and Monounsaturated fatty acids. They are considered a superfood because of their "healthy" oils that help your skin and hair stay healthy. This goes well with any smoothie you make, especially if you are going to make a fruit smoothie.

## 12.Olives

This is a great green for those who are watching their salt intake! Olives are an essential ingredient in many heart-healthy recipes that can help you lower cholesterol levels. They have also been shown to lower blood pressure and reduce inflammation.

## 13.Cucumbers

Cucumbers are a great source of water and also contain potassium, vitamin A, vitamin C and B-complex vitamins. They are perfect for any smoothie because they help to keep the smoothie cool but also add many essential nutrients!

## 14.Mushrooms

Mushrooms are a great addition to any smoothie because they aren't too strong of a flavor. They are great for adding some extra nutrients, fiber and they make you feel fuller for longer. They also contain B vitamins, selenium and Vitamin D.

## 15.Zucchinis

Zucchini is a great addition to your smoothie because it gives your smoothie a little texture and will also make your smoothie cold. Zucchinis have some great nutrients such as Vitamin C, Potassium, Magnesium, Vitamin A and Fibre. They are also loaded with water!

### 16.Squash

Squash is very similar to zucchini because of how much water it contains. Squash also contains many nutrients such as Magnesium, Vitamin A and Vitamin C. It has a very mild flavor but adds a great texture to your smoothie!

### 17.Onions

Onions add a great flavor to any smoothie! They are also a great source of Vitamin C and are very low in calorie, making them a great addition to any smoothie.

### 18.Green Bananas

Green bananas are great for adding a little texture to your smoothie. They also have many nutrients such as Vitamin C, Potassium and Fibre. They are a very mild flavor and will also make your smoothie cold!

## Nuts & Seeds

### 1.Brazil Nuts

Brazil nuts are a real treat. They contain the highest amount of selenium, a powerful antioxidant. Selenium is known to help prevent cancer. Brazil nuts also have the highest amount of pro-vitamin A in all foods, with 8,000 iu (international units) per one ounce serving. Brazil nuts are an excellent source of fiber.

### 2.Hemp Seeds

Hemp seeds are a great source of omega-3 essential fatty acids. They have the highest levels of omega-3 essential fatty acids, with about 10g per 100g serving (10 times more than salmon). The hemp seed (and all hemp products) contains very little THC, the psychoactive ingredient in marijuana. Hemp seeds are best used in smoothies and can be sprinkled over salads or cereals.

## 3.Pine Nuts

Pine nuts are a good source of omega-3 essential fatty acids and vitamin E. They are also a good source of protein and are known to be nutritious for the heart.

## 4.Sesame Seeds

Sesame seeds are high in calcium, magnesium, iron and zinc. They also contain a small amount of vitamin B1, B2, and E. They are also high in vitamin E and have more calcium than milk. Sesame seeds are very high in lignans, phytosterols that help reduce the risk of cancer and heart disease.

## 5.Pumpkin Seeds

Pumpkin seeds are a good source of essential fatty acids, zinc, and protein. They also contain a lot of iron and vitamin E. They are helpful for the prostate and are a good source of zinc, which is known to reduce the symptoms of PMS.

## 6.Walnuts

Walnuts are a good source of omega-3 essential fatty acids and vitamin E. They have the highest amount of omega-3 essential fatty acids, with about 20g in every 100g serving (20 times more than salmon). Walnuts are also a good source of protein.

## Spices

### 1.Basil

Basil has been used as a medicine since the ancient times. It is a powerful anti-fungal, antibacterial and antiseptic agent. It is useful in fighting infections especially when taken in combination with other spices like garlic, onion, turmeric and ginger. The most common form of basil is the sweet basil which has a distinctive smell. Other varieties include Thai basil that has a powerful spicy flavor and the Genovese basil that smells of cloves.

### 2.Bay Leaves

Bay leaves are dried leaves from the evergreen bay laurel shrub. It has a bitter taste and gives an aromatic flavor to soups and stews. It is used in making curry and other spicy dishes. It is also used as a remedy for headaches, dysentery, rheumatic pains and snake bites.

### 3.Cloves

Cloves are the dried flower buds of an evergreen tree native to Indonesia. The spice is used in making spicy dishes such as curry, stew and chutneys. It also has medicinal properties. It is used to treat toothache, sore throat, coughs, colds and diarrhea.

### 4.Dill Weed

Dill weed is the leafy herb of the dill plant. The herb has a strong flavor that is used in pickling vegetables and fish. It also contains essential oils such as carvone, limonene, pinene and anethol. Dill weed is also used as a remedy for flatulence and indigestion.

## 5.Parsley

Parsley is the leafy herb of a Mediterranean plant. It has an earthy flavor and contains essential oils such as apiol, myristicin and limonene. It is known to be a diuretic, preventing excessive fluid accumulations in the body. Parsley is also rich in vitamins (A, B1, B2, C and K) and minerals (iron, calcium, potassium and manganese).

## 6.Oregano

Oregano is a species of the perennial herb that is known for its strong flavor. It has been used as a remedy for respiratory problems such as asthma, coughs, colds and flu. It has also been used as an antispasmodic and anti-bacterial agent. Oregano contains vitamin A, B1, B2, C and K.

## 7.Savory

Savory is a perennial herb that is known for its aromatic flavor. It is commonly used in making stew and other spicy dishes. It also has medicinal properties including anti-spasmodic, anti-diarrhea and anti-bacterial properties.

## 8.Thyme

Thyme is a perennial flowering herb that has a strong flavor. It contains essential oils such as thymol, pinene and linalool. It is used in making soups, stews, sauces and other spicy dishes.

Thyme is also used as a remedy for coughs, colds, diarrhea and indigestion.

### 9.Sweet Basil

Sweet basil is a variety of basil that has a distinct smell. It is used in making Italian dishes and as a spice for making Italian salad dressing. It contains essential oils such as cineol, eugenol, terpineol and geraniol.

### 10.Turmeric

Turmeric is the root of an herbaceous plant native to India. It has a distinctive yellow color and pungent flavor. It has been used in Asian cuisine for centuries to make curry and other spicy dishes. Turmeric contains curcumin, which is known to have anti-inflammatory effects, anti-tumor properties and antibacterial properties.

### 11.Sage

Sage is a perennial herb that has a strong flavor. It is used in making stuffing for turkey and other poultry. It is also used for treating asthma, coughs, colds and flu.

### 12.Cayenne

Cayenne is the dried, ground fruit of a tropical plant. It has a strong peppery taste and is used in making spicy dishes such as soups, stews and chutneys. It is also used as a remedy for stomach aches, asthma, rheumatic pains and gonorrhea.

## Herbal Teas

## 1.Ginger

Ginger and turmeric are two herbs that have been used for thousands of years for their beneficial properties to the human body. Ginger has been used in the United States as an herbal medicine for stomach cramps, nausea, vomiting due to morning sickness, and diarrhea. It has also been used in China as a remedy for indigestion and heartburn. It is also a common ingredient in Chinese herbal medicine. Ginger is known for its anti-inflammatory properties, and can be helpful in reducing swelling and pain from arthritis; it can also be helpful in reducing inflammation of the joints. Ginger is also a diuretic, and is known for its ability to relieve gas in the digestive tract. It is also helpful in relieving nausea or morning sickness during pregnancy.

## 2.Fennel

Fennel is a great alternative to ginger and is also an excellent cleansing herb. It contains a natural diuretic that can help relieve gas and bloating in the gastrointestinal tract. Fennel is also known for its ability to help stimulate milk production in new mothers and has been used for centuries in India as "sweet milk tea."

## 3.Red Raspberry Leaf Tea

Drinking red raspberry leaf tea can assist women with the onset of menstruation. The tea is known for its ability to regulate blood flow by nourishing the uterus. It can also soften the cervix (the opening to the uterus) during labor which can reduce difficulty when giving birth, and reduce blood loss after childbirth. Red raspberry leaf tea is also known for its benefits in toning the reproductive organs; it is considered to be an excellent cleanser of mucous membranes (like those found in the rectum, throat, and mouth). Regular consumption of red raspberry leaves will help maintain a healthy menstrual cycle. You should drink one cup of dry red raspberry leaves steeped in one quart of boiling water at least three months prior to becoming pregnant if you want to have a healthy pregnancy, and then continue drinking two tablespoons per day during your pregnancy. You should continue drinking one cup per day after you are done nursing, in the case that you want to have more children in the future.

## 4.Chamomile Tea

Chamomile is a calming herb that is well known for its ability to relieve stress and anxiety. It has been used as a medicinal herb for centuries, and it has been found that this herb can be helpful in improving digestion and relieving irritable bowel syndrome (IBS). As an herbal tea, chamomile can assist with insomnia. In addition to its calming properties, chamomile is also known for its ability to reduce inflammation of the intestines; it has anti-inflammatory properties which can help people with inflammatory bowel syndrome (IBS) or Crohn's disease. It is also known for its anti-microbial properties which make it helpful in treating colds and flu-like symptoms.

## 5.Elderberry

Elderberry is a great herb to have on hand if you are prone to getting colds and flu. It can also be used as a preventive for the onset of seasonal allergies. Elderberry can help reduce inflammation in the respiratory system and has antiviral properties. I incorporate elderberries into my smoothies in the fall, winter, and spring.

## 6.Burdock

Burdock root is a herb that has been used in Chinese medicine for centuries. It is known for its ability to cleanse the blood and lymphatic system, and it can help detoxify the liver. Burdock root is also an effective diuretic, which can help relieve fluid retention. It contains a high amount of inulin which helps cleanse the digestive system. I use burdock in my smoothies on a regular basis, and I usually drink about one cup per day as a tea or tincture.

## Oils

### 1.Coconut Oil

Coconut Oil is a healthy fat that is found in nature and is composed of medium-chain triglycerides (MCT). Your body needs healthy fats, such as coconut oil, to function properly. Coconut Oil has a high smoke point, making it an ideal oil for cooking. When using Oils, make sure to choose organic, unrefined oils. This is great if you want your smoothie to be a little creamier.

### 2.Hemp Oil

Hemp oil is rich in omega-3 fatty acids and amino acids. Hemp seed oil contains GLA (gamma-linolenic acid), an omega-6 fatty acid. Hemp seeds are anti-inflammatory, making them a great addition to smoothies. Hemp oil is also beneficial for the immune system, heart, and skin.

### 3.Grapeseed Oil

Grapeseed Oil is a light oil with a high smoke point. Grapeseed oil has anti-inflammatory properties and is high in vitamins E and antioxidants. When choosing Oils, make sure to find one that is non-GMO and cold pressed. Your smoothie will be lighter and have a fresher flavor when you use Grapeseed Oil.

## 4.Flaxseed Oil

Flaxseed Oil is rich in omega-3 fatty acids, antioxidants, and vitamins. It also contains alpha-linolenic acid (ALA), an omega-3 fatty acid. Flaxseed oil has anti-inflammatory properties, making it beneficial for the skin and heart. When choosing Oils, make sure to find one that is non-GMO and cold pressed. Flaxseed Oil can also be added to your smoothies without being combined with another oil.

## 5.Avocado Oil

Avocado Oil is a healthy fat that is good for your heart, eyes, skin, brain, joints and digestion. Avocado Oils are rich in vitamins E and K as well as essential fatty acids (EFA's). EFAs are important for skin elasticity and help to reduce blood pressure levels in the body. When choosing Oils, make sure to find one that is non-GMO and cold-pressed. This will ensure that you get the most benefits from this healthy fat!

# Chapter 3

# Adapt Habits to Make a Difference

Habits are things we do over and over again. We don't have to think about them much in the beginning. The more we repeat a habit the stronger it becomes. If you want to change your life, you have to change your habits. The same applies to your diet and health and the Green Smoothies diet will help you to change your habits.

Making these changes will help you to achieve your goal of optimal health and well-being. You will be able to make these changes because you will already know the benefits of the Green Smoothies diet.

## Drink Lots of Water

Drinking water is essential when you are drinking Green Smoothies. Drinking lots of water will help your body to expel all the waste products that accumulate while you are transforming your body and getting rid of the toxins that are in your body.

The Green Smoothies diet is composed of lots of vegetables, fruits, and herbs. When you first start to drink Green Smoothies you may feel a little nauseous and will experience diarrhea. You will also have headaches and tiredness when you first start this diet. These symptoms are a result of your body expelling the toxins that have accumulated in your body over time. Drinking plenty of water will help with these symptoms.

Your body needs to expel these toxins and that is why the Green Smoothies diet has been formulated to be an intense detoxification program for your system. The side effects that you may experience when you start this diet are normal and are due to the cleansing process your body is going through.

Drink lots of water throughout the day so that your system gets rid of all the toxins that are in your body. Most people get headaches when they go on a detoxification program because their bodies are ridding themselves of toxins they have stored in their bodies over time. In order to have a healthy body, it is essential to drink lots of water.

When it comes to drinking water, a simple rule is to drink a glass of water every time you eat. You will find yourself drinking more and more water as you change your eating habits. The more water you drink, the more toxins you will be able to remove from your body. Drink at least six glasses of water daily.

## Say "NO" to Microwave

Drinking water is one habit that you need to make if you want to change your life. Another habit that needs to be changed is the way you prepare your meals. You need to stop using a microwave. Microwaves are very unhealthy because they cause the food to lose its nutrients and it causes the food to become harmful to your body.

A microwave will turn any type of food into a toxic substance because it uses radiation, which causes your food to become toxic. The food in a microwave is not cooked, it is "nuked" and it causes the food to become extremely harmful to your body.

Microwaves are dangerous because they cause your food to become deformed. The chemicals that are found in non-organic foods make the food taste good. However, when you burn these chemicals, they become carcinogens that will cause you to get cancer. Microwaves change the molecular structure of the natural nutrients that are found in any type of food which makes them unhealthy and toxic for your body.

Microwaves also cause your food to lose its nutritional value because most of the time these foods contain chemicals and additives that were not added by nature but by man. These additives cause problems for your body and will make you sick if you continue to eat this type of food regularly in a short period of time.

The Green Smoothies diet does not allow microwaves because microwaves make your food toxic for your body and destroy its nutritional value. When you drink Green Smoothies it is an all organic diet and does not contain any artificial or chemical ingredients. This diet makes sure that you eat healthy food instead of processed and bland foods like those found at fast-food restaurants.

When you drink Green Smoothies you are eating whole fruits and vegetables which are rich in vitamins and minerals. When you drink Green Smoothies you will feel a lot healthier and happier than when you eat fast-food meals that contain deformed, processed food that is loaded with chemicals and toxins that will make your body become sick.

# Don't Use the Word "Cheat"

If you are used to eating a certain food, it is hard to give it up. When you try to follow a new diet, it is normal to have cravings for the foods of your old diet.

The word "cheat" is not allowed on my diet and the Green Smoothies Diet. The word can make you feel guilty and that will set you back in your journey. You can always substitute your old food with a healthier food if you have a craving for one of the forbidden foods.

The reason that you are reading my book is to change your habits. You will be able to change your habits if you don't use the word "cheat" because it will set you back in your journey.

Some people have a habit of eating at night. If you are used to eating starchy foods, then you will have a craving for them at night. When you eat these foods at night, they can make it difficult for you to fall asleep.

If you have a craving for these types of foods, then eat a green smoothie instead. A green smoothie is not as satisfying as the food that you crave but it won't give you the same cravings that bread and pasta do.

If you are used to eating sweets, then try an apple or another fruit instead of sweets. You can get sweeten from fruits rather than from candies and other sugary treats. If your sweet tooth is too strong, then try making your own fruit juice without sugar and add honey. It's less sweet but if it makes the craving go away, then it is worth trying.

The point is that the word "cheat" is not allowed in my diet and if you want to change your habits, then don't use this word either. If I had told myself that I could cheat on this diet when I was first starting out with Green Smoothies, I would still be cheating on this diet because I am not a cheater. Cheaters never win in the long run.

## Have a Game Plan for Outings

When you are going on outings with friends and family, take some of your own food. You will be able to continue to enjoy these social gatherings and not feel like you have to eat what everyone else is eating.

You can also take your own food when you are on the road and traveling. You can easily carry your own food in a cooler. If you will be staying in a hotel room, make sure to take some of your own food along with you. This will save you from having to eat the foods that are available in restaurants and hotels.

You can also make it a game plan to have your own food available whenever possible. If you are eating out at a restaurant, ask the waiter or waitress if they have any items that are healthy for you to eat on their menu. You can ask for their suggestions because they know what is served at that particular restaurant. They will know what is good and nutritious for you to eat there.

If you ask other people what they think of the Green Smoothies diet, they may give you a negative response because they don't understand how this diet works. It is not just about eating green vegetables; it is about eating whole foods that are nutrient-rich and living foods that are alive with enzymes, vitamins and minerals. This type of diet gives people energy and vitality because it helps our organs function better than eating animal products and processed foods. The Green Smoothies diet helps us to maintain our natural body weight and keeps us looking younger.

## Practice Patience

You have to be patient with yourself when you are changing your habits. This is a process that takes time and you have to allow yourself enough time to make these changes. It will not take you very long to realize the benefits of the Green Smoothies diet. If you stick with it, you will feel better physically and mentally in the long term.

You should set realistic goals and give yourself some time to achieve them. You may not see immediate changes, but they will come after a few weeks of making these dietary changes. You can also make these changes in small increments so that they don't seem so overwhelming for you.

Remember, patience is a virtue, so don't become discouraged if it takes a little time for you to see results from this kind of diet change. Remember that once you start feeling better on this diet, it will motivate you even more to make more changes in your life.

For example, if you eat out a lot and order unhealthy foods, start by eating out less often and making healthier choices when you eat out. As you make healthier choices when eating out, that will make it easier for you to change your eating habits at home.

Once you start feeling better, that will motivate you to continue with these dietary changes. It is a process and the more positive changes you make in your life, the easier it will be for you to make even more positive changes.

## Plan, Plan, Plan

You need to plan your meals or snacks ahead of time. If you will be out and about, carry some snacks with you. You can take some of the Green Smoothie Recipes that we have in our book to keep you healthy wherever you are.

If you have food available for yourself whenever you are hungry, it will be easier for you to not overeat if you are eating out with friends or family. You will not feel deprived because there are many great tasting foods that can satisfy your cravings and keep your body healthy at the same time.

When you have your own food available for yourself, you will not feel like you have to eat the foods that are served at restaurants and fast food places. You can eat what you want and not have to worry about gaining weight or having health problems. This will give you freedom to make your own choices in the foods that you eat.

In addition, making these types of positive changes will help to improve your self-esteem and confidence because this is just one more step in the direction of your ultimate goal of better health and well-being.

## Prepare - A Smoothie Diet Chart

You can make a chart to keep track of how many smoothies you drink a day, your progress and the benefits you are experiencing from this diet. You will be able to see that change comes slowly at first, but as you continue to make these changes, you will see more positive results.

The chart will help you to stay focused on your goal of health and well-being. The more you follow the Green Smoothie diet, the more benefits you will see. You will feel stronger and healthier each day.

The chart should have three columns and a blank line for each day of the week. Start your chart at the top of a clean page with a heading of "Day One" and then put the next date in the next column. Then on each line, write down how many smoothies you drank during that day. The last column is to record any changes that have taken place since starting this diet. Use as many lines as you need to record these changes.

For example, if you find that you sleep better on the first day, you will write it down in the third column next to the first day. As time goes on, you will be able to see more changes taking place and your chart will help you to stay focused on your goal.

When you are finished with your chart, start a new one. Then continue with this diet until you reach your goal weight. Once you reach your goal weight, keep the chart to remind yourself of where you started and how far you have come. You will be able to see how much progress has been made and how easy it is when we make ourselves a priority in our lives.

## Stock Your Pantry for a Healthy Diet

If you want to make smoothies every day, you will need to keep some supplies on hand in your pantry. **You may want to stock up on some of the following items:**

**Green Vegetables** – Collard greens, kale, spinach and parsley are some of the most nutritious and definitely the most popular to use when making smoothies.

**Fruit** – Use fruits such as apples, grapes, oranges and berries for a hint of sweetness.

**Nuts** – Almonds, walnuts and cashews are great in smoothies to help with protein. They also add a great taste.

**Grains** – Quinoa is an excellent source of complete protein for vegetarians and can be added to any smoothie recipe that calls for nuts or seeds. Other grains such as barley are also good choices for your diet.

**Liquid** – Some of the best liquids for making green smoothies are water (filtered if possible), apple juice or grape juice if you like the taste or milk (use low-fat).

**Flavors** – Natural and artificial flavoring can add a little kick to any smoothie. One of the best natural flavorings is vanilla.

**Sweeteners** – You may want to use sweeteners such as honey or stevia in your smoothies to give a little extra sweetness without using fruits which will raise your sugar level. Stevia is an excellent natural sweetener that has no calories and no additives. This makes it an excellent choice for anyone who needs to watch their weight.

Having these things on hand will make it easy to make a smoothie anytime you feel like it. It is not hard to keep some of these things on hand in your pantry because they are the same things that you would use for your regular meals.

# Experiment with Your Food

The first thing you need to do is experiment with your diet and with the various foods that you eat. You can change some of the foods that you eat on a regular basis and replace them with some healthy fruits and vegetables. It takes time to change your habits. If you are trying to change your eating habits it may take more than a week or even a month.

In order to change a habit, you have to make one small change every day in the direction of your goal. In order for these small changes to become permanent habits, they must be repeated over and over again.

If you want to live a healthy lifestyle, then you have to make changes in all areas of your life including your personal habits, relationships, work environment and other areas of your life. Once the habit is formed in one part of your life, it will spread into other areas of your life.

Different people have different tastes and different ways of preparing food. Each person's taste buds are different and it takes time to adjust to a new diet. You should not expect to make all these changes overnight.

On average, it takes at least one month for a new habit to become permanent. You must also remember that it could take up to six months or even longer to make a permanent change. You may want to set a new goal every six months so that you can encourage yourself to continue your journey of self-discovery.

You have the power to make changes in your life. If you need help or support you may need someone who is an expert in the field of nutrition and healthy eating habits. If there is someone in your life who can help you make these changes, then you are lucky because they can help you make the right choices and provide the guidance and support you need.

Your mind has great power over everything else in your body and mind. When you think about something, it affects all areas of your life including your diet and health habits. You can use this power of thought to accomplish anything in life that you want, including achieving optimal health and well-being by changing your diet with Green Smoothies.

If there are people in your life who are against all these changes, then this will be more difficult for you but not impossible. You should try not to allow other people's opinions to affect how you live your life. You should also try to surround yourself with people who support your new healthy habits and lifestyle.

Your diet is one of the most important things you can do to improve your life. You must make these changes because they will help you to get rid of chronic problems such as constipation, headaches, arthritis and other health problems. Green Smoothies are also a great way for you to lose weight if this is an area that needs improvement in your life.

## Reward Yourself

Habits that you repeat any time at all can become bad habits. You want to reward yourself in order to help make the Green Smoothies diet a habit.

If you make the goal of drinking the Green Smoothies every day, it will be easier to stick with this habit because it is rewarding.

During the first week of the Green Smoothies diet, you will want to reward yourself every time you drink a smoothie. Treat yourself to something that is good for you and that will help to make your smoothie habit a good one.

You can also reward yourself after your first week, or at the end of each month, or after a year of drinking the Green Smoothies every day. You can treat yourself to a new book about the Green Smoothies Diet or maybe just a new pair of shoes that are healthier for your feet.

Admittedly, this is how I have been able to stick with my own healthy eating habits but it does work well. You will see results when you reward yourself in this way and it will make the Green Smoothies diet easier to stick with because it becomes rewarding for you as well as beneficial for your health.

The reason why it's so important to have a reward system is that it makes the Green Smoothies diet easier to stick with when you have something to look forward to.

When you go out and buy yourself a new pair of shoes or a new guide about the Green Smoothies Diet, then you feel happy when you make your next smoothie because you want to reward yourself for sticking to your habit. The reason why this works well is because it will make the Green Smoothies diet even more rewarding for you. The more rewarding it is for you, the more likely it is that you will stick with the Green Smoothies diet.

This is one of the time-tested methods to help make your
Green Smoothies diet more rewarding and easier to stick with.

## Track and Monitor Your Progress

Getting started with the Green Smoothies diet is easy. The
best way to track your progress is to keep a journal. A journal
will help you monitor how many times a week you drink your
green smoothie. You can also use your journal to record how
many glasses of water you drink each day or any other healthy
habits that you decide are important for you.

If you don't keep a journal, writing down these things on a
piece of paper or on a calendar will work just as well. If
keeping track of all this seems like too much work, it might be
easier to just choose one habit that seems the easiest for you
and start with that one.

Together with your Smoothie Diet Chart, you have a perfect
tool to monitor your progress and keep track of your new
habits.

For example, if you want to start with the habit of drinking
eight glasses of water a day, just write it down on your
Smoothie Diet Chart and mark it off each time you drink that
amount.

If you don't already have a smoothie diet chart, make one
now. Just take a piece of paper and write down each habit you
want to start with on the appropriate day. Some days might be
marked with more than one habit. You can either make
separate charts for each day or just add the habits to the same
chart as you go along.

If you find yourself struggling with one of your habits, just put a red X next to it or write down what is getting in the way. At the end of the week, you can look at your chart and see whether you are on track with your goal and if not, you can take corrective action.

A journal will help you to understand your challenges and how you can overcome them. Writing down what is going on inside of you makes it easier to take corrective action. You will learn from your experiences and be better prepared next time.

If you keep track of these things and find that they are too much work or that they aren't helping you, stop doing them right away. Make any changes that might be necessary so that they work for you and keep doing them until they become second nature.

It is important not to become obsessive about this because this will only hinder your progress. Just use these tools like a compass to help steer you in the right direction. Don't make it so complicated or carry it around with you all day long because that will only make it more difficult for yourself. Just use them when it is convenient for you, but do use them consistently. It is better to do too much than too little.

# Chapter 4

# Foods to Avoid

In this chapter of Dr. Sebi's book Green Smoothies, we will go into detail of the foods to avoid. He talks about the type of foods that will rid you of your health conditions and restore your youth and vitality. He continues with the types of foods that will stop your healing process. This is a very important chapter because understanding it will greatly improve your ability to stay healthy, youthful and vital. I suggest you read this chapter carefully.

We have already covered the foods that we should be eating. Now we will talk about the foods that are not recommended for consumption. These foods will cause inflammation of your organs and/or lead to illness and disease.

The foods to avoid are processed and unnatural foods, fatty meats, fried foods, refined sugars and carbohydrates (such as breads, pasta, rice etc.), dairy products (such as milk), wheat products (such as breads, pasta, crackers etc.), artificial sugars (high fructose corn syrup), additives (including salt), preservatives and colorings. This list is not exhaustive but it is a good start.

Let's take a closer look at these foods.

# Canned Fruits or Vegetables

Some people are under the impression that canned fruits or vegetables are good because they do not have preservatives. However, canned fruits contain the preservative sodium benzoate, which is a carcinogen. It converts into benzene (a known carcinogen) when it mixes with ascorbic acid (vitamin c) or vitamin B3. Ascorbic acid is added to most commercial juices in order to increase their shelf life.

So if you consume a lot of canned fruit or vegetables, then you might want to reconsider doing so. Try to get fresh fruits and vegetables from the supermarket instead of buying them from the store shelf in cans.

When you go to the supermarket, you will probably notice that fresh fruits and vegetables are usually sold near the front of the store. The fresh fruits and vegetables are usually on display. The best fruits and vegetables to buy are those that have little or no chemical residues.

Keep in mind that even though you buy something organic, it is still possible for you to experience some kind of side effects from it. This is because there could be other foods in your diet that cause a reaction when they come into contact with your organic food.

An alternative to canned fruits and vegetables is to eat frozen fruits and vegetables. Frozen fruits and vegetables are just as nutritious as fresh foods. They are processed in a way that preserves their natural nutrients, vitamins and minerals.

# Non-Vegetarian Foods

Some people eat meat and other animal products to get protein. However, these foods are hard to digest. Animal protein is also very acidic. This acidity causes your body to become acidic (which leads to cancer).

Non-vegetarian foods also contain high amounts of cholesterol and saturated fats. People who consume a lot of these meats will have an increased risk of heart disease.

If you are a non-vegetarian, then you will have to give up eating meat for a while. If you can't do this, then at least reduce the amount of meat that you are consuming each day.

The point is to avoid processed meats at all costs. It's also beneficial to reduce your consumption of non-processed meats.

## Fortified & Processed Foods

These are usually referred to as processed foods. These foods are those that have had additives, colorings, preservatives and/or chemicals added to them. Most of these foods come in boxes or cans and are loaded with fats and carbohydrates (carbohydrates come from the flour or sugar that is used to make the product).

For example, white bread is a fortified food (processed bread). This means that it has had all the nutrients removed from it. The food companies add nutrients back in after they have taken them out. How can you determine this? If you look at the ingredients on the package, you will see all sorts of chemical names such as "Enriched Flour", "Vitamin C" or "Ascorbic Acid" which is vitamin C. In addition, if you look at the nutrition label on the package, there will be a long list of ingredients used to make this product and it may contain many grams of sugar per serving.

White breads contain very little fiber. White breads are white because all the nutrients have been removed from it. It is highly processed and then fortified with chemicals to make up for the nutrients that were removed. This is why white breads are bad for you.

White flour has also been processed and then fortified back with vitamins and minerals to make up for the nutrients that were removed in the processing of the flour. In addition, white flour is bleached, which means that they use a chemical whitener to bleach the flour to give it a lighter color. Bleaching also removes all enzymes from your body, which are needed for digestion of carbohydrates (carbohydrates come from the flour).

Another example of a fortified processed food is white rice. White rice is white because all the nutrients have been removed from it in the processing. It has to be fortified with vitamins and minerals to make up for the nutrients that were removed in the processing.

So what do we do with the fortified foods? We need to avoid them. These foods have had all their nutrients removed and then added back to them. This is not a good thing.

**Let's take a look at some of the fortified foods that we should avoid:**

-White flour (breads, pasta, crackers etc.)

-White rice (white rice is white because it has been stripped of all its nutrients)

-White Sugar & High Fructose Corn Syrup

These are unnatural forms of sugar and they cause inflammation in your digestive system. They are also known to cause diabetes in many people. In addition, they can make you overweight and cause you to have high cholesterol levels. The high fructose corn syrup is found in most processed food products, such as sodas, candies, cakes, cookies, ice creams etc. You want to avoid these sugars at all costs if you want to stay healthy. It has been proven that these sugars lead to insulin resistance which leads to diabetes and obesity. Insulin resistance in turn leads to many degenerative diseases such as cancer, heart disease etc., so it is important that you avoid these sugars as much as possible especially if you already have health issues such as diabetes or obesity.

An alternative to using sugar or high fructose corn syrup is pure organic honey. You can use it in your tea or coffee instead of sugar. It is much healthier for you and will not cause the inflammation that regular sugars do.

Another alternative to using regular white sugar is stevia, which is a natural sweetener that comes from the stevia plant. You can find this sweetener in most health food stores and it comes in liquid or powder form. It has no calories, so it does not cause weight gain like regular sugar and high fructose corn syrup does. Stevia is very sweet so you only need a small amount of it to sweeten your foods. It also contains some nutrients such as iron, calcium, phosphorus etc., unlike other artificial sweeteners that have no nutrients but are loaded with chemicals like aspartame, which has been proven to cause cancer.

If you have a taste for something sweet, then try organic raw honey as your sweetener instead. The taste of raw honey is very similar to regular sugar and if you add a little cinnamon to it, then it tastes like brown sugar. Raw honey has many health benefits because its nutritional value remains intact when it is unheated (it's unheated when it is raw, unprocessed and unpasteurized).

## Dairy

The dairy industry has convinced the public that drinking milk is healthy. However, there are some things you should know about milk. In order for a calf to grow quickly, it must consume the placenta of its mother. The placenta contains hormones and proteins that will help the calf grow quickly. These same hormones and proteins (such as insulin-like growth factor) are present in human breast milk. Because of this factor, breastfeeding is recommended for infants. Cow's milk contains many hormones and proteins that will make a human infant grow quickly, which is why it can be dangerous for infants to drink cow's milk during their first year of life.

Even if you do not have an allergic reaction to cow's milk, it may still be harmful to you because it is unnatural and processed. This means that even if you do not have allergies to some of the proteins in cow's milk, they may still affect your body negatively through other mechanisms such as creating inflammation or damaging your organs over time.

The dairy industry has also convinced us that consuming lots of calcium will prevent osteoporosis as we get older. However, research has shown that increased intake of calcium may actually increase your risk of osteoporosis. This is thought to be because calcium keeps your bones hard, which makes them more prone to breakage. Soft bones are better able to withstand the bumps and falls that occur in life. Calcium helps form blood clots, which also increases the risk of heart disease, stroke and death.

If you have been drinking dairy products for most of your life (and especially if you are over the age of forty), then it may be difficult for you to stop consuming dairy products right away. If this is true for you, then I recommend you gradually reduce your intake until you can completely stop consuming it altogether (especially if you are over forty years old). If you want to do this gradually, then start by consuming less dairy on a daily basis.

In addition, the pH of dairy products is not in the alkaline range. Dairy products are in the slightly acidic range. This means that when you consume dairy products, they can make your overall diet more acidic. This may be harmful to you because your body must maintain an alkaline pH balance in order to properly digest and absorb the nutrients from your food.

## Alcohol

Dr. Sebi says alcohol is not recommended. He says alcohol is toxic and causes premature aging of the body. He says it also weakens the body's immune system and delays healing. Alcohol creates an acid condition in the body. This stops the proper function of the organs and slows down the healing process.

According to Dr. Sebi, alcohol is a poison. It is a drug. It destroys the organs and makes us age faster than we should.

Alcohol also causes many diseases such as cirrhosis of the liver, cancer, high blood pressure etc.

Drinking alcohol will only delay your healing process and it will not improve your health. If you are an alcoholic, it is important that you seriously consider stopping drinking alcohol.

One of the problems of alcohol is that it is addictive. We have already talked about how addictive sugar, wheat and dairy products are. They create a dependency on them that you will need to break. Alcohol is the same. It also creates an addiction and dependency that we must break in order to be healthy and youthful.

Drinking any type of alcohol accelerates aging and causes cancer, among other health issues. If you are able to stop drinking alcohol, then do so.

Any type of alcohol is not recommended by Dr Sebi but he seems to be more critical of distilled spirits (beer, wine, liquor). He says distilled spirits contain more harmful ingredients than beer or wine. Some people enjoy a drink now and then but it's best not to drink any alcohol if you want to stay healthy and youthful.

## Fried Foods

These are foods that have been cooked in a deep fryer. Examples of fried foods are fried chicken, French fries, fried fish etc. Fried food contains trans-fatty acids. These fatty acids cause inflammation of your organs and can lead to many degenerative diseases such as cancer, heart disease etc., so you want to avoid them at all costs.

The trans-fatty acids in fried foods also causes your body to store fat on your hips, legs and thighs more than the other areas of the body. This is because the fat cells in these areas have a greater tendency to store this type of fat. This is why you see people who have a lot of fat on their hips, legs and thighs but not much fat in their belly.

Trans-fatty acids can also cause blocked arteries and heart disease so you want to avoid them at all costs. They also cause inflammation of the arteries so that they become hard and brittle leading to plaque formation. The plaque will eventually lead to a heart attack if it is not treated properly.

It's important that while following this program you avoid fried foods at all costs. Don't eat anything that has been cooked in a deep fryer.

Fried chicken is the most common type of fried food that people consume. It should be avoided at all cost because it causes inflammation in your organs and can lead to many degenerative diseases.

Beef is also one of the most commonly consumed meats. It is also very unhealthy for you because it contains saturated fat which causes inflammation of your organs and can lead to degenerative diseases.

## Fish

Many people think that fish is healthy because it is a good protein source. However, this is a misconception. Fish has all the same characteristics as red meat. It is high in heavy metals and low in nutrients. Therefore, it should be avoided like red meat.

In addition, it is very hard to clean the fish thoroughly. Fish is also high in mercury, which can cause neurological problems such as memory loss. In addition, there are many toxic materials that fish absorb from the water that they live in.

In general, the larger the fish, the more toxic it is. So, steer clear of big fish such as tuna and swordfish. This is because they contain large amounts of heavy metals such as mercury, lead and cadmium. Fish that live in freshwater are usually safer than salt water fish.

## Soy Products

Dr. Sebi explains that soy products, such as tofu, are what he refers to as "false proteins." He says that soy products contain an enzyme blocker called "trypsin inhibitor." This enzyme inhibitor blocks the action of the enzyme trypsin and interferes with protein digestion. The enzymes contained in Dr. Sebi's green smoothies break down food into its nutrients and aid in proper digestion.

If you eat foods containing trypsin inhibitors, you will not be able to properly digest your food and it will lead to malnutrition and further illness and disease. Edamame, a Japanese dish made from boiled or steamed soybeans is not recommended because it is full of trypsin inhibitors!

He explains that if you eat tofu, which is basically just soy milk with a coagulant added, it can lead to malnutrition because the body cannot digest the proteins contained within it properly due to these enzyme blockers called trypsin inhibitors. Yogurt contains similar proteins but they are not blocked by these inhibitors so they are better tolerated by the body than tofu but they should still be avoided for optimal health!

People think that soy is good for them because certain Asian populations eat it frequently and they are often very healthy. They believe this is the reason for their good health, when really it is likely because they consume a very healthy diet and have good lifestyle habits. It's not because tofu is good for them.

He says that when Asian people move to other countries, including America, and start eating the typical American diet, they start to get sick like Americans do because their bodies are no longer accustomed to eating foods containing trypsin inhibitors. They have been eating these types of foods their whole lives so their bodies are used to them but when they eat western foods, which contain much more of these enzyme blockers, they get sick like Americans do.

This is why soy products should be avoided in order to achieve optimal health. He also mentions that even if you buy organic soy products in the health food store, which contains no pesticides or herbicides because it came from a farm that was certified organic by the USDA (United States Department of Agriculture). The USDA does not require any testing for trypsin inhibitors! This means that if you eat organic tofu or soy milk it can still be very unhealthy for you!

# Chapter 5

# Keep Keep Going After the Smoothie Cleanse

So far, we have discussed the habits and diets to get rid of with the green smoothies. The next thing is to talk about the habits and diets you need to create and practice in order to keep them. These habits are not any new ones, but they are most likely those that make it hard for you to incorporate the greens into your daily diet.

This chapter is not about creating a plan or habits. What this chapter is about is keeping the habits that will help you keep using the green smoothies and making the necessary changes that will make your green smoothies a daily habit.

## Gradually Add More Foods

Now that your body has been cleansed and is ridding itself of the junk that has accumulated for years, you must add more food. It is very important for you to add in the right foods, in the right amounts. The foods you add should be raw, unprocessed and organic. As you can see from the recipe section in this book, a small amount of cooked food can be added in.

Some people get scared by this statement, but let me assure you, it is not necessary to go cold turkey or to immediately change your diet. The transition into this new way of living will allow you to slowly make changes and continue with your daily routine without giving up everything at once. You will retain your current lifestyle and be able to gradually make changes with ease as Dr. Sebi has done for over forty years now.

It is important to eliminate meat, dairy, sugar and processed foods immediately. It is also important for you to gradually add in new foods. Adding new foods too quickly will cause you to experience certain symptoms. **Here are some of the most common symptoms you may experience when adding foods to your diet:**

-Gas, bloating and indigestion

-Constipation or diarrhea

-Headaches, achiness and fatigue

These symptoms are usually a result of food allergies that are triggered by the introduction of too many new foods at one time. It is not the foods themselves that cause these symptoms, but your body's reaction to them. In this case you should avoid these foods for two weeks and then reintroduce them one at a time to see what your body's reaction is. If you experience these symptoms after eating organic vegetables, for example, then those particular organic vegetables should be avoided for two weeks; then reintroduce them one at a time until you find out which ones cause a reaction. The same goes for fruits, nuts and seeds...you get the picture. Once you identify which foods cause any negative reactions, avoid them altogether or consume only very small amounts.

To eliminate these symptoms, just remember that the more slowly you add in new foods, the less likely you are to experience any negative reactions. **To sum up this section:**

-Get your body clean first.

-Keep all meat and animal products out of your diet.

-Add new foods one at a time, every three days or so.

For example, if you want to add quinoa, you must not eat it for three days before adding it in. Then you wait three more days and test to see if there are any negative symptoms. If there are, then stop eating quinoa for two weeks, then reintroduce it one more time and repeat the process.

## Stick to Healthy Foods

One of the most important things you can do to ensure that you're getting all of the nutrients your body needs is to stick to eating healthy, whole foods. These types of foods are packed with vitamins, minerals and fiber that will help you to feel good.

When you stick to healthy foods, you'll know that everything you are putting into your body is good for it. That's not necessarily the case with processed or packaged foods. As mentioned in the earlier chapters, processed food companies put a lot of time and effort into making sure their products taste good and look appealing. But in doing so they often take shortcuts when it comes to nutrition. They may add a lot of sugar or salt, or add ingredients that your body doesn't need.

That means that they are taking away from the nutrients that your body does need.

Your plate may look quite different if you stick with healthy food choices than if you choose processed foods. For example, you may have a salad for lunch instead of a sandwich, grilled chicken and vegetables for dinner instead of frozen pizza and fried chicken, and whole-grain cereal for breakfast instead of sugary breakfast bars.

One thing to note is that just because something is healthy doesn't mean it will taste good to you. You'll need to keep trying new foods until you find ones that make your taste buds happy. It may take some time to get used to eating healthy foods, but it will be worth it in terms of how you feel.

Sometimes, it may be tempting to just reach for any unhealthy snack food you can find. If this is something you struggle with, try storing healthy snacks around the house. Having them around will make it easier to choose them instead of the junky snacks. Also, if they are out in the open, it will be a reminder that there are healthier options available to you.

## Chew Slowly

Making sure you take time to chew your food slowly can help to ensure that you're getting the nutrients you need. When you eat quickly, you don't give yourself time to fully enjoy your food. That means that your body doesn't have time to tell you when it's satisfied.

This is important because when your body is satisfied, it naturally tells you not to eat anymore. Eating too quickly can cause you to eat more than your body needs, which leads to weight gain.

By slowing down and taking a few moments between bites, you give yourself the opportunity to fully appreciate what you are eating. This will also help lessen the temptation of eating too fast in order to get more food into your mouth before it gets cold.

For example, you might take a bite of your meal, chew it for a few moments, then take a bite of your veggies or drink some water. You don't need to spend hours chewing each bite. Just make sure you give yourself enough time to really taste what you are eating and let your body tell you when it's satisfied.

## Avoid Overeating

The best way to avoid overeating is to pay attention to your body. If you start to feel full, it is time to stop eating. One way of telling if you are full is by checking in with your stomach. It can get used to being overfilled and will feel uncomfortable when it's time to stop eating. If you have a meal or two where you eat until your stomach feels uncomfortable, the next time you sit down for a meal it will be easier for you to know when it's time to stop.

When you're hungry, you should eat. If you're not hungry, it may be a sign that your body isn't getting the nutrients it needs. The next time you feel hungry, try eating healthy foods that will help to fill your body and give it the nourishment it needs.

In addition to paying attention to your stomach, listen to other signals from your body. For example, if you feel dizzy or lightheaded after eating, that may be a sign of low blood sugar. It is important to take care of yourself and make sure this doesn't happen by keeping healthy snacks with you at all times. Other signs that you may need something more substantial include a sore throat or dry mouth. These signs could be a result of dehydration and need for fluids or perhaps an infection in the mouth. If this is the case, it is important to seek medical attention immediately as these symptoms are often warning signs for other serious medical problems.

## Hydration is the key

Your body is made up of mostly water, so it's important to keep it hydrated. If you don't, your organs will not be able to function properly and this can lead to a number of health problems, including kidney stones and kidney failure. That means you need to drink about eight ounces of water right after you wake up in the morning and before you go to bed at night.

You should also try to drink a glass of water or other healthy beverage every time you sit down for a meal. If you drink enough water throughout the day, it will help your body properly digest your foods and will help prevent constipation.

It can be difficult to remember how much water is enough if you don't drink it often. One thing that many people do is add ice cubes or lemon slices to their water to make it more interesting. This makes it easier to drink more throughout the day.

It's important to note that when you do drink water, you need to make sure it's pure and filtered. Tap or well water may contain chemicals, minerals and other substances that your body doesn't need but cannot get rid of. If you want to ensure that your water is pure, fill up a pitcher and keep it in the refrigerator. That way your water will always be at a temperature that is comfortable for drinking.

If you aren't able to consume enough water at home, try carrying around a reusable water bottle. That way you can drink some water whenever you're thirsty throughout the day. It's a good idea to have several bottles on hand so that if one gets dirty or breaks, you don't need to worry about buying a new one.

Another reason to drink water is that it will help your body to eliminate toxins and waste products. What your body doesn't need gets sent out in your urine or stool, and if your body isn't getting enough water to do this, it gets backed up. This can lead to conditions like urinary tract infections and kidney stones.

In addition, drinking enough water will help you feel full faster and for longer periods of time than if you are drinking other beverages like juice or soda pop. If you are trying to lose weight, this is important because it will prevent you from eating as many calories as when drinking liquids like juice or soda pop that contain sugar or calories from added sweeteners.

## Remember Your End Goals

Instead of focusing on the foods that you can't have, focus on the foods that you can. You don't have to constantly think about things that are off limits. Instead, focus on the things that are allowed.

It can be hard to stick to a strict diet when there is so much temptation around you. Sometimes, it may seem easier to just give in and have a piece of cake or a candy bar than it would be to deal with how bad you'll feel if you eat it. But if you remind yourself of your end goals, it can make sticking to your diet easier. And in the long run, it will make sticking with your diet worth it.

It may help to post pictures of what you want to look like or what your nutrition goals are on your fridge or other places around the house where they will remind you of why you started this diet in the first place. It can also help if family members are also involved in this diet and encourage each other along the way.

Remember that Dr. Sebi's diet and lifestyle are about so much more than just what foods you can and can't eat. It's also about the food choices you make, the supplements you take, and your overall mindset.

In fact, there are two things that you should keep in mind as you are working on your new diet. The first is to focus on what your end goals are. The second is to make sure that you have fun with it.

It may sound strange to think of a diet or lifestyle as fun, but it doesn't have to be boring or difficult. You don't have to feel like a "dieter" all of the time. Instead, try changing your perspective and recognizing that this is a lifestyle change that will help you achieve great results in many areas of your life, including health and energy levels – which will make all aspects easier for you!

Sometimes when people start a diet they feel like everything they eat is being watched by everyone they know. That can be very stressful if it means that every meal becomes an event or something that has to be planned out in detail before it happens. Instead, try focusing on making good decisions, not bad ones. You can make a decision to eat healthy foods, but then if you don't want to eat one of the options you have prepared, it's okay to have something else. Don't let it become an all-or-nothing situation, instead just focus on making good decisions as often as possible.

Be realistic about how your lifestyle changes will affect other people in your life. For example, if you are used to eating three meals a day with snacks in between, and now you are going to have five smaller meals a day instead, it could cause stress if you think that everyone else will have to change their routine too. Make sure that your family understands what is going on in your life so that they know why you need more or different types of food than before.

And don't forget about the ways that this diet can be easy and fun for you! If you like cooking or baking, try making new recipes using Dr. Sebi's ingredients and spices. You may be surprised at how delicious and satisfying they are!

# Chapter 6

# Dr. Sebi 17 Approved Alkaline Green Smoothies

## Sea Moss Apple Smoothie

**Ingredients:**

- ❑ 2 cups apple juice
- ❑ 1 tablespoon ginger
- ❑ 1 dash garlic cloves
- ❑ 2 cups ice cubes
- ❑ 1 tablespoon sea moss gel
- ❑ 1 frozen banana
- ❑ 1 dash ground cinnamon

**Nutritional facts:**

Calories: 65
Fat: 1 g
Sodium: 7 mg
Protein: 10 g
Fiber: 3 g
Carbohydrates 5 g

**Directions:**

-Take all of the ingredients, place in blender, blend until it's smooth

-When ready, serve immediately to enjoy it!

## Avocado Green Smoothie

**Ingredients:**

❏ 1 avocado, peeled and pitted

❏ 2 cups water

❏ 1 teaspoon cayenne pepper

❏ 1 teaspoon sea salt

❏ 2 cups ice cubes

❏ Juice of ½ lime (about 2 tablespoons)

**Nutritional facts:**

Calories: 92
Fat: 9 g
Sodium: 75 mg
Protein: 1 g
Fiber: 4 g
Carbohydrates: 6 g

**Directions:**

-Place all ingredients in a blender. Blend until smooth.

-Pour into glasses and serve.

## Moringa Apple Smoothie

### Ingredients:

❏ 3 cups Moringa Leaves Juice

❏ 2 cups apple juice

❏ 1 cup ice cubes

❏ 1 teaspoon vanilla extract

❏ 1 pinch sea salt

### Nutritional facts:

Calories: 224
Fat: 0 g
Sodium: 24 mg
Protein: 8 g
Fiber: 3 g
Carbohydrates 58 g

### Directions:

-Place all ingredients in a blender. Blend until smooth.

-Pour into glasses and serve.

# Cucumber Apple Smoothie

**Ingredients:**

❑ 1 cup apple juice

❑ ½ cucumber, peeled and sliced into chunks

❑ 1 teaspoon fresh ginger, grated or chopped fine

❑ 2 tablespoons flaxseed oil

❑ ½ cup ice cubes

**Nutritional facts:**

Calories: 110
Fat: 8 g
Sodium: 16 mg
Protein: 1 g
Fiber: 2 g
Carbohydrates 7 g

**Directions:**

-Place all ingredients in a blender. Blend until smooth.

-Pour into glasses and serve.

# Wild Kale Apple Smoothie

**Ingredients:**

❑ 2 cups apple juice

- ❏ 1 cup ice cubes

- ❏ Juice of 1 lime (about 2 tablespoons)

- ❏ 1 avocado, peeled and pitted

- ❏ 1 cup wild kale, chopped fine or torn into smaller pieces

## Nutritional facts:

Calories: 120
Fat: 10 g
Sodium: 59 mg
Protein: 3 g
Fiber: 3 g
Carbohydrates 5 g

## Directions:

-Place all ingredients in a blender. Blend until smooth.

-Pour into glasses and serve.

# Carrot Apple Smoothie with Ginger, Turmeric and Cardamom

## Ingredients:

- ❏ 1 cup carrot juice

- ❏ 2 cups apple juice

- ❏ Juice of 1 lime (about 2 tablespoons)

- ❏ 1 teaspoon fresh ginger, grated or chopped fine

❏ 1 pinch sea salt

❏ ½ teaspoon ground turmeric

❏ ½ teaspoon ground cardamom

❏ 1 cup ice cubes

**Nutritional facts:**

Calories: 119
Fat: 2 g
Sodium: 39 mg
Protein: 1 g
Fiber: 3 g
Carbohydrates 19 g

**Directions:**

-Place all ingredients in a blender. Blend until smooth.

-Pour into glasses and serve.

# Cucumber Lime Smoothie

**Ingredients:**

❏ 1 cucumber, peeled and sliced into chunks

❏ 1 lime, peeled and sliced into chunks

❏ 2 cups water

❏ Juice of ½ lime (about 2 tablespoons)

❑ 1 teaspoon fresh ginger, grated or chopped fine

❑ 2 tablespoons flaxseed oil

**Nutritional facts:**

Calories: 98
Fat: 9 g
Sodium: 16 mg
Protein: 1 g
Fiber: 3 g
Carbohydrates 6 g

**Directions:**

-Place all ingredients in a blender. Blend until smooth.

-Pour into glasses and serve.

## Tomato Ginger Apple Smoothie

**Ingredients:**

❑ 4 cups tomato juice

❑ 1 cup ice cubes

❑ 1 teaspoon fresh ginger, grated or chopped fine

❑ 2 tablespoons flaxseed oil

❑ Juice of ½ lime (about 2 tablespoons)

❑ 1 pinch sea salt

**Nutritional facts:**

Calories: 87
Fat: 9 g
Sodium: 21 mg
Protein: 1 g
Fiber: 3 g
Carbohydrates 5 g

**Directions:**

-Place all ingredients in a blender. Blend until smooth.

-Pour into glasses and serve.

# Avocado Strawberry Green Smoothie

**Ingredients:**

❏ 2 cups water

❏ 1 avocado, peeled and pitted

❏ 2 cups strawberries, fresh or frozen

❏ 1 tablespoon ginger, peeled and grated

❏ Juice of 1 lime (about 3 tablespoons)

**Nutritional facts:**

Calories: 83
Fat: 9 g
Sodium: 75 mg
Protein: 1 g
Fiber: 5 g

Carbohydrates 5 g

**Directions:**

-Place all ingredients in a blender. Blend until smooth.

-Pour into glasses and serve.

## Papaya Green Smoothie

**Ingredients:**

❑ 2 cups papaya, fresh or frozen

❑ 2 cups water

❑ 1 teaspoon sea salt

❑ Juice of 1 lime (about 3 tablespoons)

❑ 1 tablespoon ginger, peeled and grated

❑ 2 cups ice cubes

**Nutritional facts:**

Calories: 89
Fat: 9 g
Sodium: 75 mg
Protein: 1 g
Fiber 4 g
Carbohydrates 5 g

**Directions:**

-Place all ingredients in a blender. Blend until smooth.

-Pour into glasses and serve.

## Orange Green Smoothie With Ginger

**Ingredients:**

- 2 cups orange juice, freshly squeezed
- 1 tablespoon ginger, peeled and grated
- Juice of 1 lime (about 3 tablespoons)
- 1 tablespoon sea salt
- 2 cups ice cubes

**Nutritional facts:**

Calories: 92
Fat: 9 g
Sodium: 75 mg
Protein: 1 g
Fiber 4 g
Carbohydrates 5 g

**Directions:**

-Place all ingredients in a blender. Blend until smooth.

-Pour into glasses and serve.

# Passion Fruit Green Smoothie

## Ingredients:

❑ 2 cups passion fruit juice

❑ 1 tablespoon ginger

❑ 1 teaspoon ground cinnamon

❑ 2 cups ice cubes

## Nutritional facts:

Calories: 92
Fat: 9 g
Sodium: 75 mg
Protein: 1 g
Fiber 4 g
Carbohydrates 5 g

## Directions:

-Place all ingredients in a blender. Blend until smooth.

-Pour into glasses and serve.

# Spinach Apple Green Smoothie

## Ingredients:

❑ 2 cups apple juice

❑ 1 cup spinach, fresh

❑ 2 cups ice cubes

❑ Juice of 1 lime (about 3 tablespoons)

❑ 1 tablespoon ginger, peeled and grated

**Nutritional facts:**

Calories: 75
Fat: 9 g
Sodium: 75 mg
Protein: 1 g
Fiber 4 g
Carbohydrates 5 g

**Directions**

-Place all ingredients in a blender. Blend until smooth.

-Pour into glasses and serve.

# Raspberry Green Smoothie

**Ingredients:**

❑ 2 cups raspberries, fresh or frozen

❑ 2 cups water

❑ 1 teaspoon sea salt

❑ Juice of 1 lime (about 3 tablespoons)

❑ 1 tablespoon ginger, peeled and grated

❑ 2 cups ice cubes

**Nutritional facts:**

Calories: 89
Fat: 9 g
Sodium: 75 mg
Protein: 1 g
Fiber 4 g
Carbohydrates 5 g

**Directions:**

-Place all ingredients in a blender. Blend until smooth.

-Pour into glasses and serve.

# Celery Green Smoothie

**Ingredients:**

❑ 2 celery stalks, sliced thin (about ½ cup)

❑ 1 cucumber, peeled and chopped into pieces small enough to fit into the blender.

❑ ⅓ cup fresh parsley leaves, or 1 tablespoon dried parsley flakes

❑ 2 cups water

❑ Juice of ½ lemon (about 1 tablespoon)

**Nutritional facts:**

Calories: 26
Fat: 0 g
Sodium: 3 mg
Protein: 3 g
Fiber: 3 g
Carbohydrates 6 g

**Directions:**

-Place all ingredients in a blender. Blend until smooth.

-Pour into glasses and serve.

## Banana Celery Green Smoothie

**Ingredients:**

❑ 2 bananas, peeled and cut into pieces small enough to fit into the blender.

❑ 1 celery stick, sliced thin (about ½ cup)

❑ 1 cucumber, peeled and chopped into pieces small enough to fit into the blender.

❑ ⅓ cup fresh parsley leaves, or 1 tablespoon dried parsley flakes

❑ 2 cups water

❑ Juice of ½ lemon (about 1 tablespoon)

**Nutritional facts:**
Calories: 280

Fat: 0 g
Sodium: 3 mg
Protein: 5 g
Fiber: 6 g
Carbohydrates 69 g

**Directions:**

-Place all ingredients in a blender. Blend until smooth.

-Pour into glasses and serve.

## Grapefruit Green Smoothie

**Ingredients:**

❑ 2 cups fresh grapefruit juice (about 4 grapefruits)

❑ 1 tablespoon ginger, peeled and chopped fine

❑ 1 dash garlic cloves

❑ 2 cups ice cubes

❑ 1 tablespoon sea moss gel

❑ 1 frozen banana

❑ 2 tablespoons flax seeds

**Nutritional facts:**

Calories: 161
Fat: 4 g
Sodium: 8 mg
Protein: 2 g

Fiber: 5 g
Carbohydrates 34 g

**Directions:**

-Take all of the ingredients, place in a blender, blend until it's smooth.

-When ready, serve immediately to enjoy it!

# Conclusion

We have come to the end of this book and I'm sure you are just as excited as I am. We have discussed how to make Dr. Sebi Green Smoothies, what they can do for you, and we have gone over a few recipes. You now have the knowledge of Dr. Sebi Green Smoothies and how to use them to your advantage. As a whole, this book has been organized in a way that will allow you to get the information you need easily.

I hope that I have been able to help you get on the road to better health with these green smoothies. As I mentioned before, my intention was not for this book to be merely informative but also instructional in nature. If you follow all of the instructions exactly as they are written in this book then there is no doubt in my mind that your health will improve dramatically. This is an extremely powerful program and is one of nature's most effective remedies.

As they say, "Live a long life and live it well!"

I have given you all of the information that I could think of and you will be able to see just how powerful green smoothies can be if used properly. I have also offered a few recipes for you to try, but do not stop there. Don't let this book collect dust and add nothing more than a few recipes. This is an incredible program that has been around for decades, read the book, use it, apply it, and watch your health improve. It may not happen overnight but I guarantee that you will see results with continued use.

Remember that you are what you eat and you are what you think. "Change your diet and change your life!"

I sincerely hope that you are able to use this information to better your health and I wish you the best of luck.

# Thank You

Thank you for buying my book and I hope you enjoyed it. If you found any value in this book I would really appreciate it if you'd take a minute to post a review about this book. I check all my reviews and love to get feedback.

# Other Books By Author

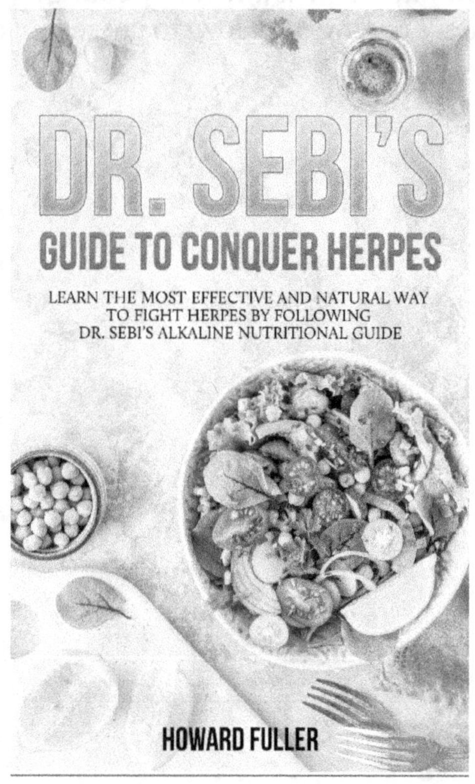

**Dr. Sebi's Guide To Conquer Herpes:**

**Learn the Most Effective and Natural Way to Fight Herpes by Following Dr. Sebi's Alkaline Nutritional Guide**

# About Author

Howard Fuller is a college dietitian graduate who was healed from diabetes and high blood pressure after changing his dietary lifestyle to Dr. Sebi Alkaline Diet. Over the years in his career, Howard found himself very unhappy by one size fits all dietary approaches and seemingly one way road towards curing diseases.

Since then, he has been inspired to research and write about Dr. Sebi's natural way of healing. He loves cooking and writing about the wonder of natural health and herbal remedies. He has written many books deepening and expanding what is already a wealth of knowledge. He is passionate and truly loves what he does and is driven by the success he has of helping others achieve.